USING HERBS FOR MEDICINE

EASY TO FOLLOW DIRECTIONS ON HOW TO USE HERBS FOR MEDICINE

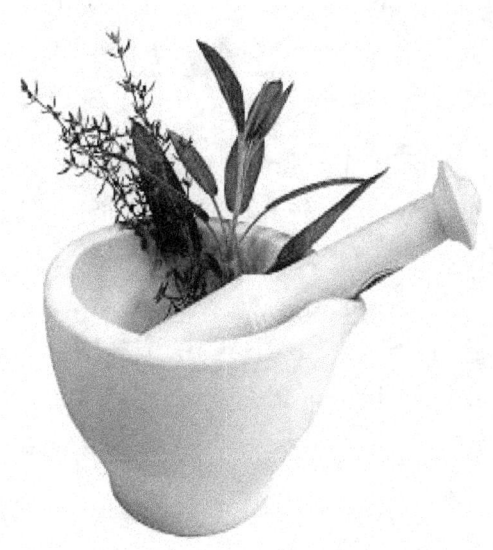

By Beverly Hill

Introduction

I want to thank you and congratulate you for choosing the book, *"USING HERBS FOR MEDICINE: Easy to Follow Direction on How to Use Herbs for Medicine"*. This book contains proven steps and strategies on how herbs are used for medicine and maintaining good health.

In a day and age of increased awareness of "living healthy," attention has naturally turned to the use of whole foods as part of a healthy lifestyle. More and more people are reducing the use of processed foods and instead focusing on natural foods – in their whole form. As part of this process, it seems inevitable that those in search of a healthier lifestyle turn their attention to using herbs for health.

It's no secret that herbs have been used for centuries to enhance food, increase and sustain health, and remedy a host of ailments. Since prehistoric times herbs for health have been part of the human experience. And as more and more herbs were discovered to have healing principles, herbs for health were soon organized into a classification system that allowed people to take full advantage of their properties in food and medicine.

Thanks again for choosing this book, I hope you enjoy it!

ABOUT THE AUTHOR

Beverly Hill is a sociologist. She is the CEO of C.E.F Associates and formerly served as head of department of sociology in Premier Natural Resources Inc.

A graduate of Nelson High School also graduated from the University of Toronto with a B.A in economics and finance and holds an M.S from Cambridge University in public relations and PhD in sociology.

She has written many articles on human equality, animal rights, environmental issues, personal development and peace keeping in different newspapers. She has also appeared in many magazines and is frequently interviewed for articles on family, race, socioeconomic status, and how to survive in your environment. She has also worked on the importance of health of relationship between parents and children. Her book 'The Middle Child' focuses on the importance of the attention given to the children and what to expect from them. This book helps parents understand their children.

In addition to these works she is also the author of 'Surviving Alone ' which is about her own childhood growing up; she writes about her family struggles living on a low income budget and growing her own food to survive.

C.E.F Associates formed in 1999 in Idaho, USA she worked both nationally and internationally. This is a consulting company which has clients all over the world. Ms. Hill the CEO of the company is the main reason of the huge client base because of her servings in foreign countries.

TABLE OF CONTENT

Chapter 1

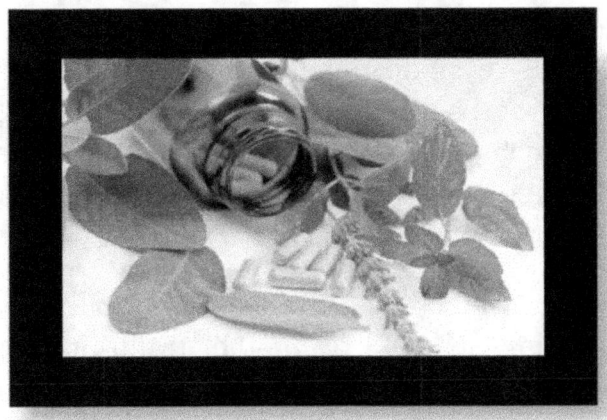

WHAT IS HERBAL MEDICINE

Herbs have played a major part in medicine for thousands of years. Every culture and every medicinal system, from Ayurveda to Traditional Chinese Medicine, have used herbs for therapeutic purposes. There are thousands of herbs with thousands of different uses, many of which are used in conventional medicine, as well as for natural remedies.

Herbs are widely used today, in teas, vitamins and natural supplements. While the benefits of herbal medicine are vast, it is important to understand the basis of herbal medicine, and to recognize that some herbs can have negative impacts on health.

WHAT IS THE HISTORY OF HERBAL MEDICINE?

Herbal medicine has its roots in every culture around the world, from the Greeks, to the Celts, the Romans to the Arabs, and the Chinese to the Indians.

Western herbalism dates back to ancient Egypt, where records of garlic and juniper used for medicinal purposes were found from as early as 1700 B.C. By 100 B.C., the Greeks had developed a comprehensive philosophy of herbal medicine that related different herbs to different temperaments, seasons, and elements such as earth, air, fire and water. The Romans took the Greek theories of medicine and added to them, creating a wealth of medical practices, some of which are still used today.

Eastern herbalism mainly comes from the traditions of Ayurveda and Traditional Chinese Medicine (TCM). These two medicinal systems use herbs to bring the body back in balance so that it can heal itself. In TCM, this means restoring qi, or "life energy," an balancing the yin forces with the yang forces. Both traditions incorporate knowledge of the elements, the seasons, and parts of the body into their herbal treatments.

Other traditions such as Native Americans from both North America and South America have used herbs in medicine. Many of these traditions incorporate ritual and magic into their practices with the use of a shaman, or medicine man.

THE PRINCIPLES OF HERBAL MEDICINE

Herbalism is designed to use herbs to treat the underlying causes of disease in a client. Instead of looking at the signs and symptoms, and then treating the disease, herbalists look at the whole picture, from lifestyle to physical stressors, in order to prescribe the right treatment.

Once the cause of a condition is discovered, the herb is prescribed to restore the body's natural balance. Herbalism understands how different herbs work with the body to restore balance and health.

Herbs are also used in many traditions as a preventative action to boost immune function, and promote general wellbeing before any disease occurs.

While many pharmaceutical companies use the active ingredients found in herbs in their products, herbalists believe in something called "herbal synergy," which means that in order for the herb to be as safe and effective as possible, it is important to use the whole plant instead of extracting only the active ingredients. For instance, meadowsweet contains salicylic acid, which is the active ingredient in aspirin. While aspirin alone often causes issues in people who have sensitive stomachs, meadowsweet also contains tannin and mucilage, which work to protect the stomach from the salicylic acid.

DIFFERENT TYPES OF HERBAL MEDICINE

There are many different types of herbal medicine with roots in many different traditions. For more information on different medicinal systems that use herbs, see Ayurveda and Traditional Chinese Medicine.

PREPARING HERBS

Decoctions are made by boiling barks, roots and berries to extract the active ingredients. The liquid is strained, and can be taken either hot or cold.

Tinctures are made by soaking herbs in water and alcohol to extract and preserve the active ingredients. The liquid is then stored in small bottles, and taken with water.

Infusions are made like teas. Boiling water is poured over the herb, and is left to sit for about 10 minutes, creating a liquid to be taken as a hot drink or medicine.

Infused Oils are made with chopped herbs and oil. The mixture is either placed in a bowl over boiling water, or left to infuse in the sunlight.

Creams are made from herbs and either oil or fat. The mixture simmers for about three hours before it is strained, and set in dark bottles.

Ointments are also made from herbs combined with either oil or fat. The ointment is then heated quickly over boiling water before it is strained and set.

BENEFITS OF HERBL MEDICINE

Herbal medicine can be very useful for treating many different illnesses from minor scrapes to burns to serious diseases. Herbal medicines are mostly used for persistent illnesses such as migraines, arthritis, depression, and PMS.

NOTE: Herbal remedies are easy to take, and many herbs can be grown at home, so they are often more convenient for minor conditions. It is important to note that herbal remedies cannot replace conventional treatments in many cases, and that not all herbs are safe for human ingestion.

Chapter 2

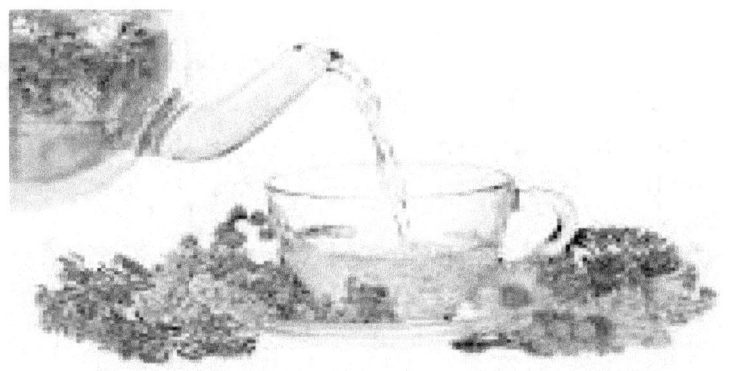

SOME COMMONLY USED HERBS

1. **Echinacea** – often used in tinctures or powders to reduce symptoms of the common cold and flu. It is also used for infections, particularly those of the kidney.

2. **Garlic** – used to reduce cholesterol levels and blood pressure, as well as for treating infections. It can be taken fresh, as a powder, as oil, or as a juice.

3. **Ginger** – commonly used to reduce nausea, to reduce symptoms of colds and chills through sweating, and to boost circulation. It can be taken fresh, dried, or as oil.

4. **Gingko** – most commonly used to improve memory. Gingko improves circulation, particularly to the brain, though it is also used to regulate irregular heartbeats, and to reduce symptoms of dementia. It is usually taken as a tincture or an infusion.

5. **Ginseng** – used to boost the immune system and decrease fatigue. It is also used for lungs conditions

such as cough, and to reduce blood pressure. The root is taken as a powder, tincture, or decoction.

6. **St. John's Wort** – used as an anti-depressant, for anxiety, irritability and exhaustion. It can also be used topically for burns and inflammations. St. John's Wort is usually taken as an infusion, tincture or scream.

7. **Lavender** – popular as aromatic oil, and can be used to treat a wide variety of ailments from exhaustion to headaches, and indigestion to depression. It is commonly taken as an infusion, tincture, mouthwash, cream, lotion, massage oil, chest rub, hair rise, or oil.

8. **Chamomile** – a popular herb used for indigestion, stress relief, anxiety, and insomnia. It is also used for asthma and bronchitis. It can be taken as an infusion, tincture, ointment, inhalation, or mouthwash.

Many people use herbs as daily supplements, or to treat specific ailments. While it usually safe and effective to do so, it is important to educate your-self on the correct way to use each herb, as some are not safe to ingest. If you do decide to take an herbal supplement, it is important to let your health care provider know, as many herbs interact with other forms of medicine.

Chapter 3

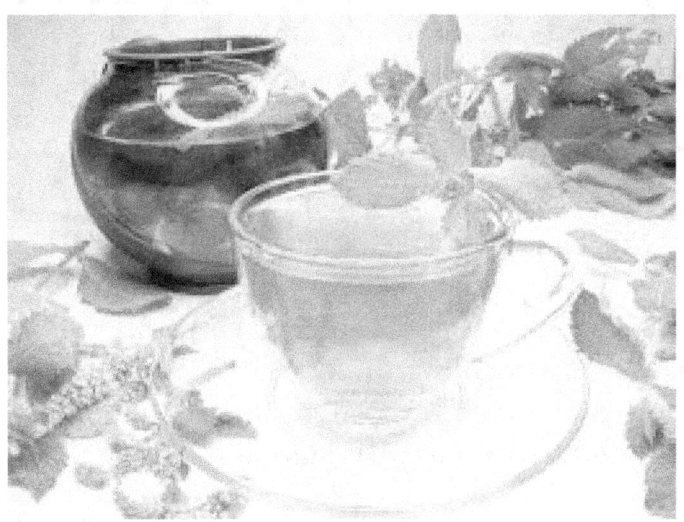

HISTORY BEHIND USING HERBS FOR MEDICINE

Man has always used herbs for medicine. From the beginning of time this practice has been documented. The first instance was in ancient Egypt when garlic, juniper and myrrh were used to ward off infections and general disease turns out that they were definitely onto something, as garlic consistently tops the charts in terms of having antibiotic, and healing properties.

This type of medical and herbal healing was used as early as 1500BC. Then, later on, in about 1000AD medical writings in England were found, and the content was mostly about how herbs could be used to help people who were suffering from various diseases. Having said that, the knowledge of herbs was also not very advanced back then, as most doctors thought that disease came from being shot at with eleven arrows!

Luckily, human theory – with regard to health and medicine – advanced, and by the twelfth century, people had taken the work of Hippocrates into account, and started believing that the solution for great health was more in line with good diet and exercise. At this time, herbs were still used for treatment of all sorts of ailments and affections. Herbs were also used in an effort to prevent poor health in general. Shortly after the twelfth century, the church decreed that certain herbs had been signed by God, and practitioners were heavily encouraged to make use of them in their treatments. They would group the herbs according to color. The white herbs would be used to treat mothers who were breastfeeding, and the yellow herbs would be used to treat jaundiced patients.

Then, as medical knowledge advanced, and as printing presses became available, herbalists would start to spread the word about their creations, and people from all over the world got to experience the power of this shared knowledge. There was a definite improvement in the general health of people over this period of time, as there could be a lot of discussion about what works, and does not in terms of a herbal remedy.

Herbal medicine rose to real prominence again in the 19th century, when a botanist who was disenchanted by medicine at the time decided to heal people through the use of roots and herbs. This approach formed the basis for modern day homeopathy.

HERBS IN MODERN MEDICINE

Today, we use herbs in conjunction with western medicine to achieve optimum results. This is called integrated medicine and it recognizes the fact that there are some ailments that western medicine cannot treat as well as herbs can – and vice versa. Herbs are also sometimes used to stave off the side effects of western medicine which can often be devastating to the body when used in large, consistent doses.

Chapter 4

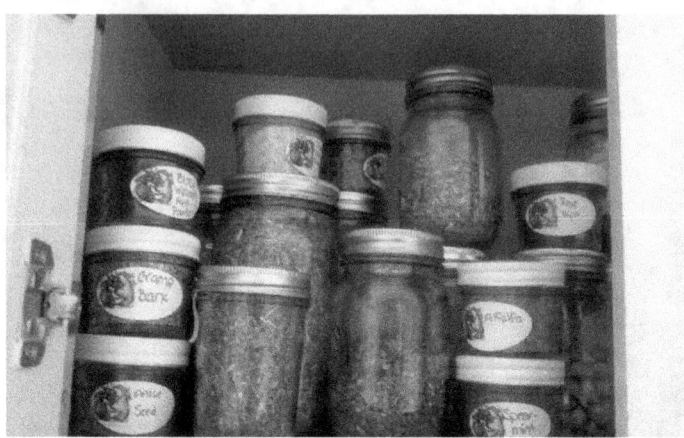

TIPS FOR DRYING HERBS FOR MEDICINAL USE

The way you harvest and dry your herbs depends greatly on what your planned usages is for the herbs are. There are a few general rules that should be followed; however, if you are planning on using the herbs for medicinal, culinary, or aromatic reasons. Remember if you are drying herbs to use in floral arrangements to be particularly careful of the flowers.

The best time to collect and harvest any herb is in the morning after any dew as dried in the sun. The time of year will greatly depend upon the use. If you are looking for the scent of a particular herb, you want to snip the leaves before the herb flowers. If you are looking for the flowers to harvest, you want to cut them before they actually bloom. The drying process will not impede the actual opening of the bloom. For seeds, you want to collect them before they crack open, and fall off to propagate.

There are several methods of drying whatever the part of the herb you are looking to use. A simple method that works is to lay a screen out in a dry sunny location, and place the stems of herb in a single layer across it. Turn the herbs at least once a day until they are dry. Don't have a screen cover a baking sheet with a double layer of paper towel and lay the herbs on it, works just as well.

If you are harvesting a large quantity of herbs, you may wish to use a different method than the screen. One way is to tie up the stems with a rubber band (the herb stems will shrink as they dry), and hang them in a warm dark location with plenty of air movement. If you have a dust issue try poking holes in a brown paper bag, and place over the herbs (be careful not to touch the flowers), and hang for about two weeks.

Drying seeds wrap a brown paper bag (no holes this time) around the stems of the herb, and hang the bag so that the seeds will fall into the bottom of the bag. It will take about two weeks for all the seeds to fall.

Need the herbs dried now. There is always the oven. Spread a single layer of herbs on a cookie sheet and place in the oven (set the oven on the lowest possible temperature setting). Leave the oven on and turn the herbs at least once a day (twice is better). They will be dry (depending on the type of herb) within hours.

Chapter 5

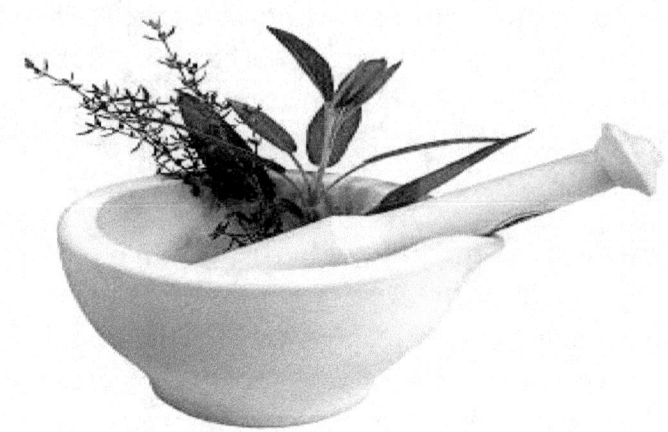

HOW TO USE HERBS FOR MEDICINE

Although herbs and vitamins can help one after becoming ill, the best and most efficient use of them is as a preventative. This means you need to take them before you become sick, on a regular, ongoing basis. Many people just can't stand the idea of swallowing pills, drinking liquid herbal extracts, etc..But that's something you need to overcome in order to maintain optimal health, and stop yourself from becoming sick in the first place.

Another thing I hear is that people believe it's too expensive to buy the good products at health food stores. Thank about it. What's more expensive in the long run, buying supplements on a regular basis, and taking them daily, or becoming ill, and in some cases, very ill? Invest in your health, and take it seriously.

Before taking anything though, do your research. A lot of people, for instance, don't understand how to use herbs, or vitamins safely for the best results. Did you know that your body can build up immunity to Echinacea? Echinacea should be used in a rotation of thirty days at a time, then stopped for thirty days, then restarted for another thirty days. The best time to start using it (in my opinion) is about the first of October, stop for November, and restart in December. And take it as directed on the package. Don't skip doses. Herbs are always best in the form of a liquid tincture. The dry herb capsules are never as potent, because most of the oil in them has evaporated. But they're better than nothing.

As far as vitamins are concerned, many people also don't understand that you can take very large amounts of certain vitamins, particularly vitamin C, with absolutely no harmful side effects, and a great benefit. Vitamin C is one of those vitamins that your body will simply eliminate any excess of that it can't use. The same goes with most B vitamins, but doing your research is important. Vitamin A in the form of Beta-carotene is not the same as regular Vitamin A, because Beta-carotene is water-soluble, whereas Vitamin A in its oil-based form is not. Which means you can take large doses of beta-carotene safely, but not so for Vitamin A.

I can't stress enough the importance of using supplements as a preventative. So many people will come down with a cold, and THEN started wolfing down the vitamin C, which won't hurt but won't provide you with what you're looking for. It really is a lifestyle choice, no different than exercising, and eating a good diet. And I truly don't believe you can get the optimal amount of vitamins and minerals from diet alone. I've used herbs and vitamins, amino acids, all kinds of things, for over twenty years now. And I can attest, from personal experience that they can work very well as a preventative.

Chapter 6

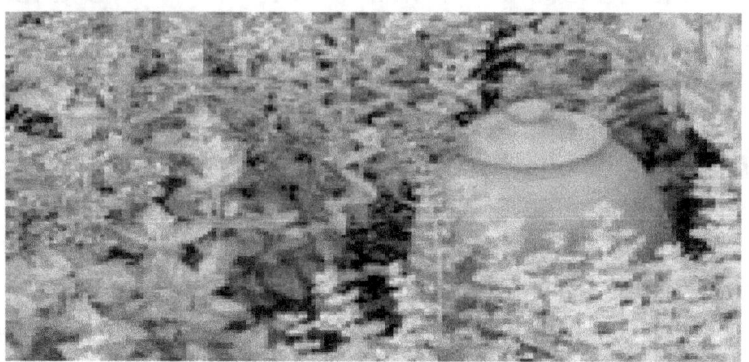

HERB GARDEN FOR MEDICINAL PURPOSE

Herbs are fantastic plants which are well known for the fragrance, flavor, medicinal and cooking qualities. Many people use them for cooking, as medicines, and even spiritually when using the herbs for medicine or spiritual purposes the roots are often used. Many of the culinary herbs are leafy and green full of flavor and texture. Some plants can be used as a spice and an herb, such as dill or coriander, and others are simply grown as an herb.

Throughout history herbs have been used for their medicinal purposes, and some herbs that are used in very small doses will do well, but in large doses can kill. You must ensure that you know what you are doing when selecting the herbs to treat someone with. Chinese medicine is world famous for the use of herbs, and these doctors have studied for many years to fully understand the qualities and benefits of every herb available.

Herbs can become a part of your everyday life; not only are they fantastic to grow to eat with but also many smell fantastic when growing. Certain herbs such as mint and peppermint are great to have to deter pests such as flies, and mice. When you have these herbs growing the pest won't enter your home, and the herbs are perfectly safe around children and pets. You will find that if you are growing herbs then you will add them to many different dishes that you are cooking. You will find that they add great flavors too many different meals, and you will never cook without them in the future.

Growing your own herb garden is very easy; you will find that the more you nurture your crops the more they will flourish. Picking them at the right time is essential, and if you are not aiming to pick them for that day then you can freeze dry the herbs. Drying them is a great way to ensure that none of your herb garden goes to waste, and then you can enjoy them even out of season. Deciding what to plant in your herb garden will be entirely up to choice. You may want to start small, and only plant a couple of herbs, and as you get more experienced then you can increase your herb collection.

You will need to consider how each of the herbs grows, and what their habits are; if some need more sunlight than others this can affect all of them. Choosing your herbs wisely will ensure that you get the best from your herbs. If you go to a reputable garden center they will be able to advise which herbs would suit your garden, and which ones will grow well together. Once you begin growing your own herbs you will never go back to shop buying them again. You will find that your grown ones will taste fresher, and nicer, and be much easier to use. If you are very interested in herbs there are several websites and books available, which will look at the history, and medicinal purpose of herbs.

Conclusion

Thank you again for choosing this book!

I hope this book was able to help you to see how herbs can help with simple illnesses, and can work very well as a preventative.

Using herbs for health can be as convenient and as simple as you make it. An array of natural herbs can be found as close as your local grocery store; as well as in farmers markets and health foods stores. But for those who want herbs at their fingertips for a variety of uses, it may be beneficial to plant your own herb garden.

Either way, a little bit of research will have an enormous amount of information about the uses of herbs for health. With some planning and simple integration of herbs into your everyday routine, you may be surprised at how your overall health and vitality begins to improve.

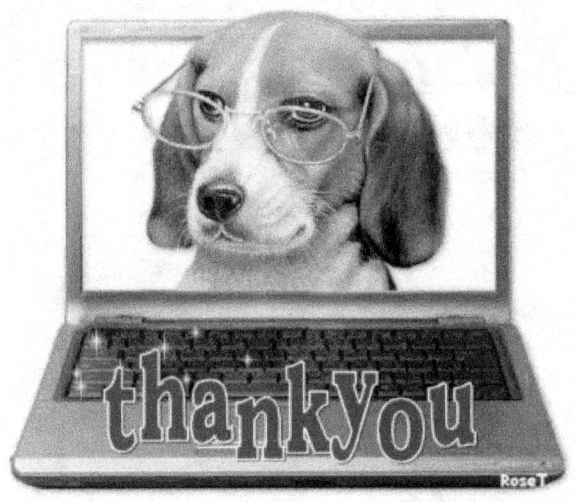

Finally, if you enjoyed this book, would you be kind enough to leave a review for this book on Amazon? It'd be greatly appreciated!

Thank you and good luck!

Preview Of 'HERBAL GARDENING: HOW TO GROW YOUR OWN HERBS INDOORS AND OUTDOORS'

Chapter 1

HERBAL GARDENING

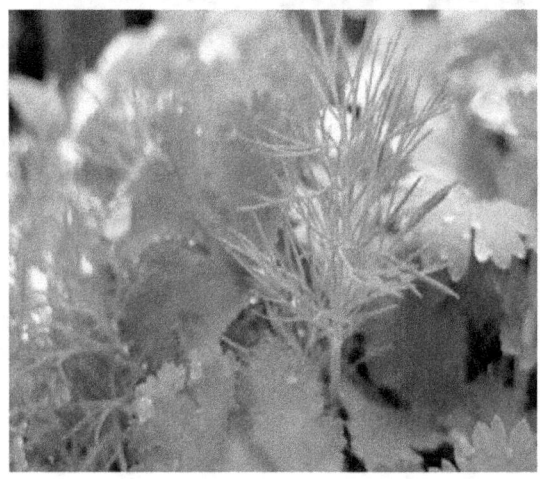

Herbs are very easy to grow with a little sunshine, soil that drains well, some watering, and a little fertilizer or compost. Herbs can be grown in pots: however, the plants always prefer to be in the ground where they can spread out. Some plants grow quite large (4-6 feet), and when placed in pots they can become stunted and can get stressed, which causes them to be very unhappy. Main Thing Necessary to Grow Herbs is to put them in the Right Place.

The main requirement for growing Herbs is growing them in the proper location. Most prefer full sun as long as regular summer temperatures don't rise above 90 degrees. If you have very warm summers, then consider planting in an area that gets morning sun and afternoon shade in the summertime, or a place that receives filtered light (such as under a tree that allows some light to pass through). Check the area several times during the day to make sure that there are at least four hours of sun. (e.g., 8 to 12, 12 to 4, or from 9 to 11 and 2 to 4)

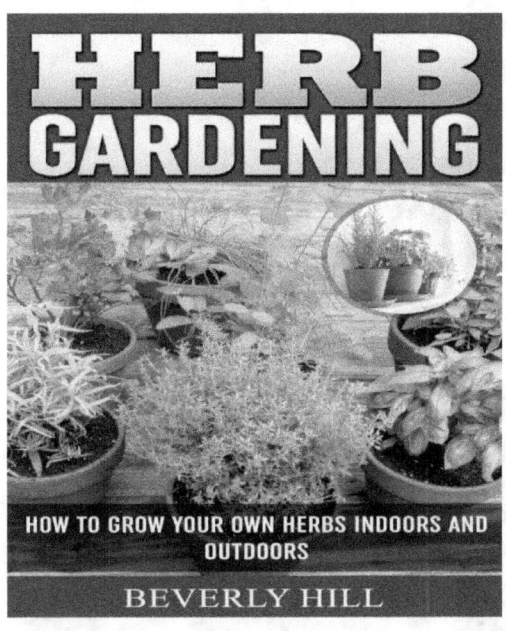

To check out the rest of (HERB GARDENING: HOW TO GROW YOUR OWN HERBS INDOORS AND OUTDOORS) go to Amazon.com

Check Out My Other Books

Below you'll find some of my other popular books that are popular on Amazon and Kindle as well. Alternatively, you can visit my author page on Amazon to see other work done by me.

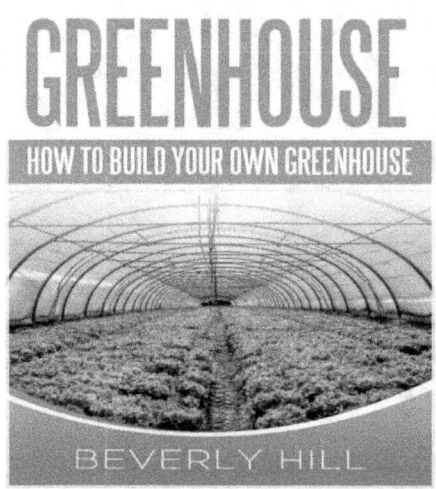

GREENHOUSE: HOW TO BUILD YOUR OWN GREENHOUSE

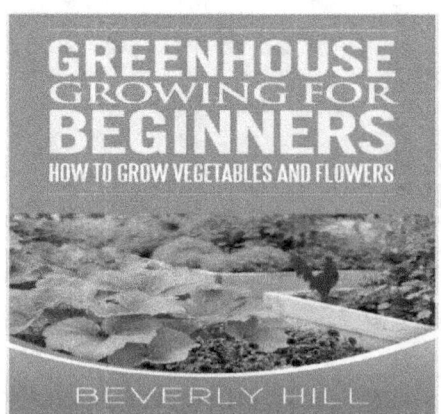

GREENHOUSE GROWING FOR BEGINNERS: HOW TO GROW VEGETABLES AND FLOWERS.

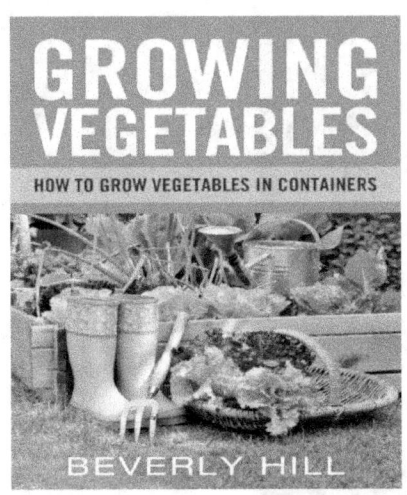

GROWING VEGETABLES: HOW TO GROW VEGETABLES IN CONTAINERS.

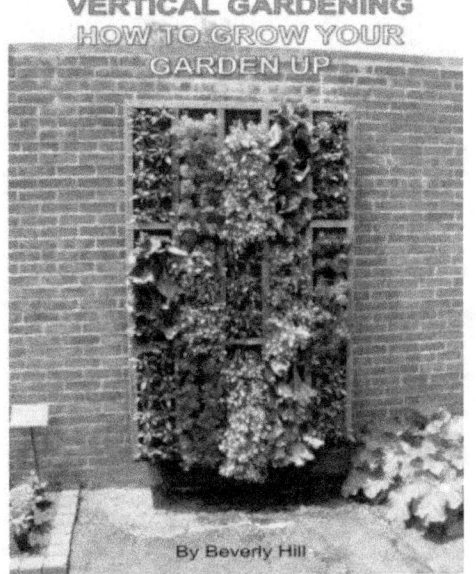

VIRTICAL GARDENING: HOW TO GROW YOUR GARDEN UP.

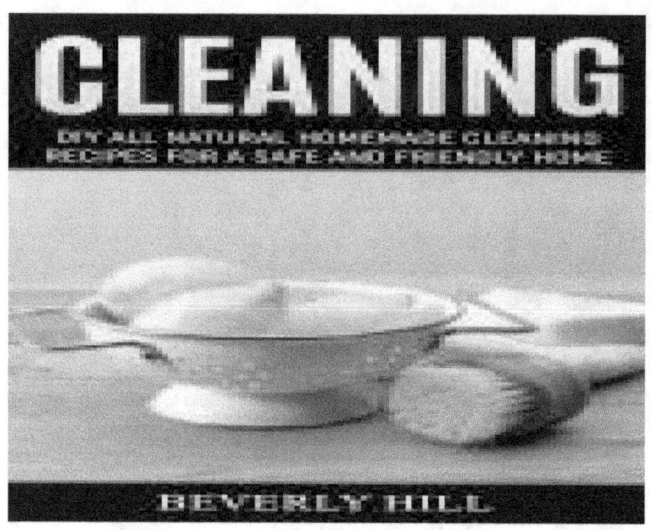

CLEANING: DIY ALL NATURAL HOMEMADE CLEANING RECIPES FOR A SAFE AND FRIENDLY HOME.

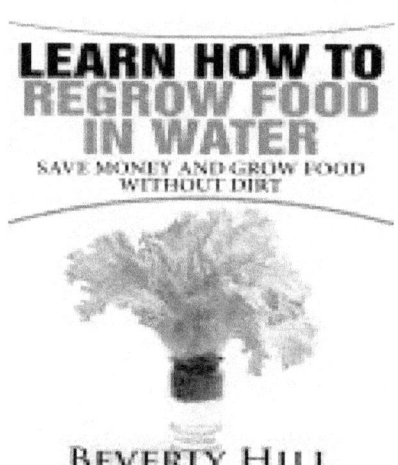

LEARN HOW TO REGROW FOOD IN WATER: SAVE MONEY AND GROW FOOD WITHOUT DIRT.

BONUS: SUBSCRIBE TO THE FREE BOOK

Beginners Guide to Yoga & Meditation

"Stressed out? Do You Feel Like The World Is Crashing Down Around You? Want To Take A Vacation That Will Relax Your Mind, Body And Spirit? Well this Easy To Read Step By Step

E-Book Makes It All Possible!"

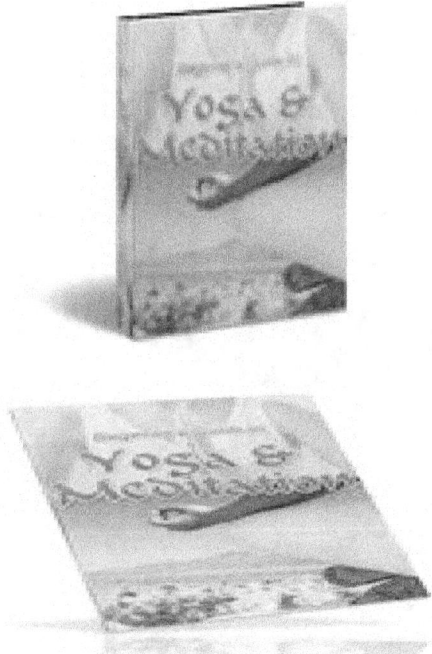

Instructions on how to join our mailing list, and receive a free copy of "Yoga and Meditation" can be found in any of my Kindle eBooks.

NOTES

NOTES

NOTES

NOTES

NOTES

NOTES